# A Defence of Free-Thinking in Mathematics

In answer
To a Pamphlet of *Philalethes Cantabrigiensis*, intituled,
*Geometry no Friend to Infidelity, or a Defence of Sir
ISAAC NEWTON, and the BRITISH Mathematicians.*
Also an Appendix concerning Mr. WALTON's
Vindication of the Principles of Fluxions contained in the
ANALYST

by

George Berkeley

I. When I read your Defence of the *British* Mathematicians, I could not Sir, but admire your Courage in asserting with such undoubting Assurance things so easily disproved. This to me seemed unaccountable, till I reflected on what you say (*P.* 32.) when upon my having appealed to every thinking Reader, whether it be possible to frame any clear Conception of Fluxions, you express your self in the following manner, "Pray sir who are those thinking Readers you appeal to? Are they Geometricians or Persons wholly ignorant of Geometry? If the former I leave it to them: if the latter, I ask how well are they qualified to judge of the Method of Fluxions?" It must be acknowledged you seem by this Dilemma secure in the favour of one Part of your Readers, and the ignorance of the other. I am nevertheless persuaded there are fair and candid Men among the Mathematicians. And for those who are not Mathematicians, I shall endeavour so to unveil this Mystery, and put the Controversy between us in such a Light, as that every Reader of ordinary Sense and Reflection may be a competent Judge thereof.

II. You express an extreme Surprize and Concern, "that I should take so much Pains to depreciate one of the noblest Sciences, to disparage and traduce a Set of learned Men whose Labours so greatly conduce to the Honour of this Island (*P.* 5), to lessen the Reputation and Authority of Sir *Isaac Newton* and his Followers, by shewing that they are not such Masters of Reason as they are generally presumed to be; and to depreciate the Science they profess, by demonstrating to the World, that it is not of that Clearness and certainty as is commonly imagined." All which, you insist, "appears very strange to you and the rest of that famous University, who plainly see of how great Use Mathematical Learning is to Mankind." Hence you take occasion to declaim on the usefulness of Mathematics in the several Branches, and then to redouble your Surprize and Amazement (*P.* 19 and 20). To all which Declamation I reply that it is quite beside the Purpose. For I allow, and always have allowed, its full claim of Merit to whatever is useful and true in the Mathematics: But that which is not so, the less it employs Men's time and thoughts, the better. And after all you have said or can say, I believe the unprejudiced Reader will think with me, that things obscure are not therefore sacred; and that it is no more a Crime, to canvass and detect unsound Principles or false Reasonings in Mathematics, than in any other Part of Learning.

III. You are, it seems, much at a loss to understand the Usefulness or Tendency or Prudence of my Attempt. I thought I had sufficiently explained this in the *Analyst*. But for your further Satisfaction shall here tell you, it is very well known, that several Persons who deride Faith and Mysteries in Religion, admit the Doctrine of Fluxions for true and certain. Now if it be shewn that Fluxions are really most incomprehensible Mysteries, and that those, who believe them to be clear and scientific, do entertain an implicite Faith in the Author of that Method; will not this furnish a fair *Argumentum ad Hominem* against Men, who reject that very thing in Religion which they admit in humane Learning? And is it not a proper Way to abate the Pride, and discredit the Pretensions of those, who insist upon clear Ideas in Points of Faith, if it be shewn that they do without them even in Science?

IV. As to my timing this Charge; why now and not before, since I had published Hints thereof many Years ago? Surely I am obliged to give no Account of this: If what hath been said in the Analyst be not sufficient; suppose that I had not Leisure, or that I did not think it expedient, or that I had no Mind to it. When a Man thinks fit to publish any Thing, either in Mathematics, or in any other Part of Learning; what avails it, or indeed what Right hath any one to ask, why at this or that Time; in this or that Manner; upon this or that Motive? Let the Reader judge, if it suffice not, that what I publish is true, and that I have a Right to publish such Truths, when and how I please in a free Country.

V. I do not say, that Mathematicians, as such, are Infidels; or that Geometry is a Friend to Infidelity, which you untruly insinuate, as you do many other Things; whence you raise Topics for invective: But I say there are certain Mathematicians, who are known to be so; and that there are others, who are not Mathematicians, who are influenced by a Regard for their Authority. Some perhaps, who live in the University, may not be apprised of this; but the intelligent and observing Reader, who lives in the World, and is acquainted with the Humour of the Times, and the Characters of Men, is well aware, there are too many that deride Mysteries, and yet admire Fluxions; who yield that Faith to a mere Mortal, which they deny to *Jesus Christ*, whose Religion they make it their Study and Business to discredit. The owning this is not to own, that Men who reason well, are Enemies to Religion, as you would represent it: On the contrary, I endeavour to shew, that such men are defective in Point of Reason and Judgement, and that they do the very Thing they would seem to despise.

VI. There are, I make no doubt, among the Mathematicians many sincere Believers in *Jesus Christ*; I know several such my self; but I addressed my Analyst to an Infidel; and on very good Grounds, I supposed that besides him, there were other Deriders of Faith, who had nevertheless a profound Veneration for Fluxions; and I was willing to set forth the Inconsistence of such Men. If there be no such Thing as Infidels, who pretend to Knowledge in the modern Analysis, I own my self misinformed, and shall gladly be found in a Mistake; but even in that Case, my Remarks upon Fluxions are not the less true; nor will it follow, that I have no Right to examine them on the Foot of Humane Science, even though Religion were quite unconcerned, and though I had no End to serve but Truth. But you are very angry (*P.* 13 *and* 14.) that I should enter the Lists with reasoning Infidels, and attack them upon their Pretensions to Science: And hence you take Occasion to shew your Spleen against the Clergy. I will not take upon me to say, that I know you to be a Minute Philosopher your self: But I know, the Minute Philosophers make just such Compliments as you do to our Church, and are just as angry as you can be at any, who undertake to defend Religion by Reason.

If we resolve all into Faith, they laugh at us and our Faith: And if we attempt to Reason, they are angry at us: They pretend we go out of our Province, and they recommend to us a blind implicite Faith. Such is the Inconsistence of our Adversaries. But it is to be hoped, there will never be wanting Men to deal with them at their own Weapons; and to shew, they are by no Means those Masters of Reason; which they would fain pass for.

VII. I do not say, as you would represent me, that we have no better Reason for our Religion, than you have for Fluxions: but I say, that an Infidel, who believes the Doctrine of Fluxions, acts a very inconsistent Part, in pretending to reject the Christian Religion, because he cannot believe what he doth not comprehend; or because he cannot assent without Evidence; or because he cannot submit his Faith to Authority. Whether there are such Infidels, I submit to the Judgement of the Reader. For my own Part I make no Doubt of it, having seen some shrewd Signs thereof my self, and having been very credibly informed thereof by others. Nor doth this Charge seem the less credible, for your being so sensibly touched, and denying it with so much Passion. You, indeed, do not stick to affirm, that the persons who informed me are *a pack of base profligate and impudent liars* (*P.* 27). How far the Reader will think fit to adopt your passions I cannot say; but I can truly say, the late celebrated Mr. *Addison* is one of the persons, whom you are pleased to characterize in those modest and mannerly terms. He assured me that the Infidelity of a certain noted Mathematician, still living, was one principal reason assigned by a witty man of those times for his being an Infidel. Not, that I imagine Geometry disposeth men to Infidelity; but that from other causes, such as Presumption, Ignorance, or Vanity, like other Men Geometricians also become Infidels, and that the supposed light and evidence of their science gains credit to their Infidelity.

VIII. You reproach me with "Calumny, detraction, and artifice" (*P.* 15). You recommend such means as are "innocent and just, rather than the criminal method of lessening or detracting from my opponents" (*ibid.*). You accuse me of the "*odium Theologicum*, the intemperate Zeal of Divines," that I do "*stare super vias antiquas*," (*P*. 13.) with much more to the same effect. For all which charge I depend on the reader's candour, that he will not take your word, but read and judge for himself. In which case he will be able to discern (though he should be no Mathematician) how passionate and unjust your reproaches are, and how possible it is, for a man to cry out against Calumny and practise it in the same breath. Considering how impatient all mankind are when their prejudices are looked into, I do not wonder to see you rail and rage at the rate you do. But if your own Imagination be strongly shocked and moved, you cannot therefore conclude, that a sincere endeavour to free a science, so useful and ornamental to Humane Life, from those subtilties, obscurities, and paradoxes which render it inaccessible to most men, will be thought a criminal undertaking by such as are in their right mind. Much less can you hope that an illustrious Seminary of Learned men, which hath produced so many free-spirited inquirers after Truth, will at once enter into your passions and degenerate into a nest of Bigots.

IX. I observe upon the Inconsistency of certain Infidel Analysts. I remark some defects in the principles of the modern Analysis. I take the liberty decently to dissent from Sir *Isaac Newton*. I propose some helps to abridge the trouble of Mathematical studies and render them more useful. What is there in all this that should make you declaim on the usefulness of practical Mathematics? that should move you to cry out *Spain, Inquisition, Odium Theologicum*? By what figure of Speech, do you extend, what is said of the modern Analysis, to Mathematics in general, or what is said of Mathematical Infidels to all Mathematicians, or the confuting an errour in Science to burning or hanging the Authors? But it is nothing new or strange, that men should choose to indulge their passions, rather than quit their opinions how absurd soever. Hence the frightful visions and tragical uproars of

Bigoted men, be the Subject of their Bigotry what it will. A very remarkable instance of this you give (*P. 27*) where, upon my having said that a deference to certain Mathematical Infidels, as I was credibly informed, had been one motive to Infidelity, you ask with no small emotion, "For God's sake are we in *England* or in *Spain*? Is this the language of a Familiar who is whispering an Inquisitor, *&c*?" And the page before you exclaim in the following Words. "Let us burn or hang up all the Mathematicians in *Great Britain*, or halloo the mob upon them to tear them to pieces every Mother's son of them, *Tros Rutulusve fuat*, Laymen or Clergymen, *&c*. Let us dig up the bodies of Dr. *Barrow* and Sir *Isaac Newton*, and burn them under the Gallows," *&c*.

X. The Reader need not be a Mathematician, to see how vain all this tragedy of yours is. And if he be as thoroughly satisfied as I am, that the cause of Fluxions cannot be defended by reason, he will be as little surprised as I am, to see you betake your self to the arts of all bigoted men, raising terrour and calling in the passions to your assistance. Whether those Rhetorical flourishes about the Inquisition and the Gallies are not quite ridiculous, I leave to be determined by the Reader. Who will also judge (though he should not be skilled in Geometry) whether I have given the least grounds, for this and a World of such like declamation? and whether I have not constantly treated those celebrated Writers, with all proper respect, though I take the liberty in certain points to differ from them?

XI. As I heartily abhor an Inquisition in Faith, so I think you have no right to erect one in Science. At the time of writing your defence you seem to have been overcome with Passion: But now you may be supposed cool, I desire you to reflect whether it be not wrote in the true spirit of an Inquisitor. Whether this becomes a Person so exceeding delicate himself upon that Point? And whether your Brethren the *Analysts* will think themselves honoured or obliged by you, for having defended their Doctrine, in the same manner as any declaiming Bigot would defend

Transubstantiation? The same false colours, the same intemperate Sallies, and the same Indignation against common Sense!

XII. In a matter of mere Science, where authority hath nothing to do, you constantly endeavour to overbear me with authorities, and load me with envy. If I see a Sophism in the writings of a great Author, and, in compliment to his understanding, suspect he could hardly be quite satisfyed with his own demonstration: This sets you on declaiming for several pages. It is pompously set forth, as a criminal method of detracting from great men, as a concerted project to lessen their reputation, as making them pass for imposters. If I publish my free thoughts, which I have as much right to publish as any other man, it is imputed to rashness and vanity and the love of opposition. Though perhaps my late publication, of what had been hinted twenty five years ago, may acquit me of this charge in the eyes of an impartial Reader. But when I consider the perplexities that beset a man, who undertakes to defend the doctrine of Fluxions, I can easily forgive your anger.

XIII. Two sorts of learned men there are: one, who candidly seek Truth by rational means. These are never averse to have their principles looked into, and examined by the test of Reason. Another sort there is who learn by *route* a set of principles and a way of thinking which happen to be in vogue. These betray themselves by their anger and surprise, whenever their principles are freely canvassed. But you must not expect, that your Reader will make himself a party to your passions or your prejudices. I freely own that Sir *Isaac Newton* hath shew'd himself an extraordinary Mathematician, a profound Naturalist, a Person of the greatest Abilities and Erudition. Thus far I can readily go, but I cannot go the lengths that you do. I shall never say of him as you do, *Vestigia pronus adoro* (*P.* 70). This same adoration that you pay to him, I will pay only to Truth.

XIV. You may, indeed, your self be an Idolater of whom you please: But then you have no right to insult and exclaim at other men, because they do not adore your Idol. Great as Sir *Isaac Newton* was, I think he hath, on more occasions than one, shew'd himself not to be infallible. Particularly, his demonstration of the Doctrine of Fluxions I take to be defective, and I cannot help thinking that he was not quite pleased with it himself. And yet this doth not hinder but the method may be useful, considered as an art of Invention. You, who are a Mathematician, must acknowledge, there have been divers such methods admitted in Mathematics, which are not demonstrative. Such, for instance, are the Inductions of Doctor *Wallis* in his Arithmetic of Infinites, and such, what *Harriot* and, after him, *Descartes* have wrote concerning the roots of affected Æquations. It will not, nevertheless, thence follow that those methods are useless; but only, that they are not to be allowed of as Premises in a strict Demonstration.

XV. No great Name upon earth shall ever make me accept things obscure for clear, or Sophisms for Demonstrations. Nor may you ever hope to deter me from freely speaking what I freely think, by those arguments *ad invidia* which at every turn you employ against me. You represent your self (*P.* 52) as a man, "*whose highest ambition is in the lowest degree to imitate Sir* Isaac Newton." It might, perhaps, have suited better with your appellation of *Philalethes*, and been altogether as laudable, if your highest ambition had been to discover Truth. Very consistently with the character you give of your self, you speak of it as a sort of crime (*P.* 70) to think it possible, you should ever "*see further, or go beyond Sir* Isaac Newton." And I am persuaded you speak the Sentiments of many more besides your self. But there are others who are not afraid to sift the Principles of human Science, who think it no honour to imitate the greatest man in his Defects, who even think it no crime to desire to know, not only beyond Sir *Isaac Newton*, but beyond all mankind. And whoever thinks otherwise, I appeal to the Reader, whether he can properly be called a Philosopher.

XVI. Because I am not guilty of your mean Idolatry, you inveigh against me as a person conceited of my own Abilities; not considering that a person of less Abilities may know more on a certain point than one of greater; not considering that a purblind eye, in a close and narrow view, may discern more of a thing, than a much better eye in a more extensive prospect; not considering that this is to fix a *ne plus ultra*, to put a stop to all future inquiries; Lastly, not considering that this is in fact, so much as in you lies, converting the Republick of Letters into an absolute monarchy, that it is even introducing a kind of Philosophic Popery among a free People.

XVII. I have said (and I venture still to say) that a Fluxion is incomprehensible: That second, third and fourth Fluxions are yet more incomprehensible: That it is not possible to conceive a simple Infinitesimal: That it is yet less possible to conceive an Infinitesimal of an Infinitesimal, and so onward.[1] What have you to say in answer to this? Do you attempt to clear up the notion of a Fluxion or a Difference? Nothing like it; you only "assure me (upon your bare word) from your own experience, and that of several others whom you could name, that the Doctrine of Fluxions may be clearly conceived and distinctly comprehended; and that if I am puzzled about it and do not understand it, yet others do." But can you think, Sir, I shall take your word when I refuse to take your Master's?

XVIII. Upon this point every Reader of common sense may judge as well as the most profound Mathematician. The simple apprehension of a thing defined is not made more perfect by any subsequent progress in Mathematics. What any man evidently knows, he knows as well as you or Sir *Isaac Newton*. And every one can know whether the object of this method be (as you would have us think) clearly conceivable. To judge of this, no depth of Science is requisite, but only a bare attention to what

---

[1] *Analyst*, Sect. 4, 5, 6, &c.

passes in his own mind. And the same is to be understood of all definitions in all Sciences whatsoever. In none of which can it be supposed, that a man of Sense and Spirit will take any definition or principle on trust, without sifting it to the bottom, and trying how far he can or he cannot conceive it. This is the course I have taken and shall take, however you and your Brethren may declaim against it, and place it in the most invidious Light.

XIX. It is usual with you to admonish me to look over a second time, to consult, examine, weigh the words of Sir *Isaac*. In answer to which I will venture to say, that I have taken as much pains as (I sincerely believe) any man living, to understand that great Author and to make sense of his principles. No industry nor caution nor attention, I assure you, have been wanting on my part. So that, if I do not understand him, it is not my fault but my misfortune. Upon other subjects you are pleased to compliment me with depth of thought and uncommon abilities, (*P*. 5 and 84.) But I freely own, I have no pretence to those things. The only advantage I pretend to, is that I have always thought and judged for my self. And, as I never had a master in Mathematics, so I fairly followed the dictates of my own mind in examining, and censuring the authors I read upon that subject, with the same freedom that I used upon any other; taking nothing on trust, and believing that no writer was infallible. And a man of moderate parts, who takes this painful course in studying the principles of any Science, may be supposed to walk more surely than those of greater abilities, who set out with more speed and less care.

XX. What I insist on is, that the idea of a Fluxion simply considered is not at all improved or amended by any progress, though ever so great, in the Analysis: neither are the demonstrations of the general rules of that method at all cleared up by applying them. The reason of which is, because in operating or calculating, men do not return to contemplate the original principles of the method, which they constantly presuppose, but are employed in working, by notes and symbols, denoting the Fluxions supposed to have been at first explained, and according to rules supposed to have been at first demonstrated. This I say to encourage those, who are not far gone in these Studies, to use intrepidly their own judgement, without a blind or a mean deference to the best of Mathematicians, who are no more qualified than they are, to judge of the simple apprehension, or the evidence of what is delivered in the first elements of the method; men by further and frequent use or exercise becoming only more accustomed to the symbols and rules, which doth not make either the foregoing notions more clear, or the foregoing proofs more perfect. Every Reader of common sense, that will but use his faculties, knows as well as the most profound Analyst what idea he frames or can frame of Velocity without motion, or of motion without extension, of magnitude which is neither finite nor infinite, or of a quantity having no magnitude which is yet divisible, of a figure where there is no space, of proportion between nothings, or of a real product from nothing multiplied by something. He need not be far gone in Geometry to know, that obscure principles are not to be admitted in Demonstration: That if a man destroys his own Hypothesis, he at the same time destroys what was built upon it: That errour in the premises, not rectified, must produce errour in the conclusion.

XXI. In my opinion the greatest men have their Prejudices. Men learn the elements of Science from others: And every learner hath a deference more or less to authority, especially the young learners, few of that kind caring to dwell long upon Principles, but inclining rather to take them upon trust: And things early admitted by repetition become familiar: And this familiarity at length passeth for Evidence. Now to me it seems, there are certain points tacitly admitted by Mathematicians, which are neither evident nor true. And such points or principles ever mixing with their reasonings do lead them into paradoxes and perplexities. If the great author of the fluxionary method were early imbued with such notions, it would only shew he was a man. And if by vertue of some latent errour in his principles a man be drawn into fallacious reasonings, it is nothing strange that he should take them for true: And, nevertheless, if, when urged by perplexities and uncouth consequences, and driven to arts and shifts, he should entertain some doubt thereof, it is no more than one may naturally suppose, might befall a great genius grappling with an insuperable difficulty: Which is the light in which I have placed Sir *Isaac Newton*.[2] Hereupon you are pleased to remark, that I represent the great author not only as a weak but an ill man, as a Deceiver and an Impostor. The Reader will judge how justly.

XXII. As to the rest of your colourings and glosses, your reproaches and insults and outcries, I shall pass them over, only desiring the Reader not to take your word, but read what I have written, and he will want no other answer. It hath been often observed that the worst cause produceth the greatest clamour, and indeed you are so clamorous throughout your defence that the Reader, although he should be no Mathematician, provided he understands common sense and hath observed the ways of men, will be apt to suspect that you are in the wrong. It should seem, therefore, that your Brethren the Analysts are but little obliged to you, for this new method of declaiming in Mathematics. Whether they are more obliged by your Reasoning I shall now examine.

XXIII. You ask me (*P*. 32) where I find Sir *Isaac Newton* using such expressions as the Velocities of Velocities, the second, third, and fourth Velocities, &c. This you set forth as a pious fraud and unfair representation. I answer, that if according to Sir *Isaac Newton* a Fluxion be the velocity of an increment, then according to him I may call the Fluxion of a Fluxion the Velocity of a Velocity. But for the truth of the antecedent see his introduction to the Quadrature of Curves, where his own words are, *motuum vel incrementorum velocitates nominando Fluxiones*. See also the second Lemma of the second Book of his mathematical principles

---

[2] *Analyst,* Sect. 18.

of natural Philosophy where he expresseth himself in the following manner, *velocitates incrementorum ac decrementorum quas etiam, motus, mutationes & fluxiones quantitatum nominare licet.* And that he admits Fluxions of Fluxions, or second, third, fourth Fluxions, *&c.* see his Treatise of the Quadrature of Curves. I ask now, Is it not plain, that if a Fluxion be a Velocity, then the Fluxion of a Fluxion may agreeably thereunto be called the Velocity of a Velocity? In like manner if by a Fluxion is meant a nascent augment, will it not then follow, that the Fluxion of a Fluxion or second Fluxion is the nascent augment of a nascent augment? Can anything be plainer? Let the Reader now judge who is unfair.

XXIV. I had observed, that the Great Author had proceeded illegitimately, in obtaining the Fluxion or moment of the Rectangle of two flowing quantities; and that he did not fairly get rid of the Rectangle of the moments. In answer to this you alledge, that the errour arising from the omission of such rectangle (allowing it to be an errour) is so small that it is insignificant. This you dwell upon and exemplify to no other purpose, but to amuse your Reader and mislead him from the Question; which in truth is not concerning the accuracy of computing or measuring in practice, but concerning the accuracy of the reasoning in science. That this was really the case, and that the smallness of the practical errour no wise concerns it, must be so plain to any one who reads the Analyst, that I wonder how you could be ignorant of it.

XXV. You would fain persuade your Reader, that I make an absurd quarrel against errours of no significancy in practice, and represent Mathematicians as proceeding blindfold in their approximations, in all which I cannot help thinking there is on your part either great ignorance or great disingenuity. If you mean to defend the reasonableness and use of approximations or of the method of Indivisibles, I have nothing to say. But then you must remember this is not the Doctrine of Fluxions: it is none of that

Analysis with which I am concerned. That I am far from quarrelling at approximations in Geometry is manifest from the thirty third and fifty third Queries in the Analyst. And that the method of Fluxions pretends to somewhat more than the method of indivisibles is plain; because Sir *Isaac* disclaims this method as not Geometrical.[3] And that the method of Fluxions is supposed accurate in Geometrical rigour is manifest, to whoever considers what the Great Author writes about it; especially in his Introduction to the Quadrature of Curves where he saith *In rebus mathematicis errores quam minimi non sunt contemnendi.* Which expression you have seen quoted in the Analyst, and yet you seem ignorant thereof, and indeed, of the very end and Design of the Great Author in this his invention of Fluxions.

XXVI. As oft as you talk of finite quantities inconsiderable in practice Sir *Isaac* disowns your apology. *Cave*, saith he, *intellexeris finitas.* And, although Quantities less than sensible may be of no account in practice, yet none of your masters, nor will even you your self venture to say, they are of no account in Theory and in Reasoning. The application in gross practice is not the point questioned, but the rigour and justness of the reasoning. And it is evident that, be the subject ever so little, or ever so inconsiderable, this doth not hinder but that a person treating thereof may commit very great errours in Logic, which Logical errours are in no wise to be measured by the sensible or practical inconveniences thence arising, which, perchance may be none at all. It must be owned, that after you have misled and amused your less qualified Reader (as you call him) you return to the real point in controversy, and set your self to justifie Sir *Isaac*'s method of getting rid of the abovementioned Rectangle. And here I must intreat the Reader to observe how fairly you proceed.

XXVII. First then you affirm (*P*. 44), "that, neither in the Demonstration of the Rule for finding the fluxion of the

---

[3] *See the Scholium at the end of the first section.* Lib. i., Phil. Nat. Prin. Math.

rectangle of two flowing quantities, nor in anything preceding or following it, is any mention so much as once made of the increment of the rectangle of such flowing quantities." Now I affirm the direct contrary. For in the very passage by you quoted in this same page, from the first case of the second lemma of the second Book of Sir *Isaac*'s principles, beginning with *Rectangulum quodvis motu perpetuo auctum*, and ending with *igitur laterum incrementis totis* a and b *generatur rectanguli incrementum aB + bA*. Q.E.D. In this very passage I say is express mention made of the increment of such Rectangle. As this is matter of fact, I refer it to the Reader's own eyes. Of what rectangle have we here the Increment? is it not plainly of that whose sides have *a* and *b* for their *incrementa tota*, that is, of *AB*. Let any Reader judge whether it be not plain from the words, the sense, and the context, that the Great Author in the end of his demonstration understands his *incrementum* as belonging to the *Rectangulum quodvis* at the beginning. Is not the same also evident from the very lemma it self prefixed to the Demonstration? The sense whereof is (as the author there explains it) that if the moments of the flowing quantities *A* and *B* are called *a* and *b*, then the *momentum vel mutatio geniti rectanguli AB* will be *aB + bA*. Either therefore the conclusion of the demonstration is not the thing which was to be demonstrated, or the *Rectanguli incrementum aB + bA* belongs to the rectangle *AB*.

XXVIII. All this is so plain that nothing can be more so; and yet you would fain perplex this plain case by distinguishing between an increment and a moment. But it is evident to every one, who has any notion of Demonstration, that the *incrementum* in the conclusion must be the *momentum* in the Lemma; and to suppose it otherwise is no credit to the Author. It is in effect supposing him to be one who did not know what he would demonstrate. But let us hear Sir *Isaac*'s own words: *Earum (quantitatum scilicet fluentium) incrementa vel decrementa momentanea sub nomine momentorum intelligo*. And you observe your self that he useth the word *moment* to signify either an increment or decrement. Hence with an intention to puzzle me you propose the increment and decrement of *AB*, and ask which of these I would call the moment? The case you say is difficult. My answer is very plain and easy, to wit, Either of them. You, indeed, make a different answer, and from the Author's saying that, by a moment he understands either the momentaneous increment or decrement of the flowing quantities, you would have us conclude, by a very wonderful inference, that his moment is neither the increment nor decrement thereof. Would it not be as good an inference, Because a number is either odd or even, to conclude it is neither? Can any one make sense of this? Or can even your self hope that this will go down with the Reader, how little soever qualified? It must be owned, you endeavour to obtrude this inference on him, rather by mirth and humour than by reasoning. Your are merry, I say, and (*P.* 46) represent the two mathematical quantities as pleading their rights, as tossing up cross and pile, as disputing amicably. You talk of their claiming preference, their agreeing, their boyishness and their gravity. And after this ingenious digression you address me in the following words —-Believe me there is no remedy, you must acquiesce. But my answer is that I will neither believe you nor acquiesce; there is a plain remedy in common sense; and to prevent surprise I desire the Reader always to keep the controverted point in view, to examine your reasons, and be cautious how he takes your word, but most of all when you are positive or eloquent or merry.

XXIX. A page or two after, you very candidly represent your case to be that of an ass between two bottles of hay: it is your own expression. The cause of your perplexity is that you know not, whether the velocity of *AB* increasing or of *AB* decreasing is to be esteemed the Fluxion, or proportional to the moment of the rectangle. My opinion, agreeably to what hath been premised, is that either may be deemed the Fluxion. But you tell us (*P.* 49) "that you think, the venerable ghost of Sir *Isaac Newton* whispers you, the Velocity you seek for is neither the one nor the other of these, but is the velocity which the flowing rectangle hath, not while it is greater or less than *AB*, but at that very instant of time that it is *AB*." For my part, in the rectangle *AB* considered simply in it self, without either increasing or diminishing, I can conceive no velocity at all. And if the Reader is of my mind, he will not take either your word, or even the word of a Ghost how venerable soever, for velocity without motion. You proceed and tell us that, in like manner, the moment of the rectangle is neither it's increment or decrement. This you would have us believe on the authority of his Ghost, in direct opposition to what Sir *Isaac* himself asserted when alive. *Incrementa* (saith he) *vel decrementa momentanea sub nomine momentorum intelligo: ita ut incrementa pro momentis addititiis seu affirmativis, ac decrementa pro subductitiis seu negativis habeantur.*[4] I will not in your style bid the Reader believe me, but Believe his eyes.

XXX. To me it verily seems, that you have undertaken the defence of what you do not understand. To mend the matter, you say, "you do not consider *AB* as lying at either extremity of the moment, but as extended to the middle of it; as having acquired the one half of the moment, and as being about to acquire the other; or, as having lost one half of it, and being about to lose the other." Now, in the name of Truth, I entreat you to tell what this moment is, to the middle whereof the rectangle is extended? This moment, I say, which is acquired, which is lost, which is cut in two, or distinguished into halfs? Is it a finite quantity, or an infinitesimal, or a mere limit, or nothing at all? Take it in what sense you will, I cannot make your defence either consistent or intelligible. For if you take it in either of the two former senses, you contradict Sir *Isaac Newton*. And if you take it in either of the latter, you contradict common sense; it being plain, that what hath no magnitude, or is no quantity, cannot be divided. And here I must entreat the reader to preserve his full freedom of mind intire, and not weakly suffer his judgment to be overborn by your

---

[4] Princip. Phil. Nat. Lib. II, Lem. II.

imagination and your prejudices, by great names and authorities, by Ghosts and Visions, and above all by that extreme satisfaction and complacency with which you utter your strange conceits; if words without a meaning may be called so. After having given this unintelligible account, you ask with your accustomed air, "What say you Sir? Is this a just and legitimate reason for Sir *Isaac*'s proceeding as he did? I think you must acknowledge it to be so." But alas! I acknowledge no such thing. I find no sense or reason in what you say. Let the Reader find it if he can.

XXXI. In the next Place (*P.* 50) you charge me with want of caution. "Inasmuch (say you) as that quantity which Sir *Isaac Newton* through his whole Lemma, and all the several Cases of it, constantly calls a *Moment*, without confining it to be either an increment or decrement, is by you inconsiderately and arbitrarily, and without any Shadow of Reason given, supposed and determined to be an increment." To which Charge I reply that it is as untrue as it is peremptory. For that, in the foregoing citation from the first case of Sir *Isaac*'s Lemma, he expressly determines it to be an Increment. And as this particular Instance or Passage was that which I objected to, it was reasonable and proper for me to consider the Moment in that same Light. But take it increment or decrement as you will, the Objections still lie and the Difficulties are equally insuperable. You then proceed to extoll the great Author of the fluxionary Method, and to bestow some *Brusqueries* upon those who unadvisedly dare to differ from him. To all which I shall give no answer.

XXXII. Afterwards to remove (as you say) all Scruple and Difficulty about this affair, you observe that the Moment of the Rectangle determined by Sir *Isaac Newton*, and the Increment of the Rectangle determined by me are perfectly and exactly equal, supposing $a$ and $b$ to be diminished *ad infinitum*: and for proof of this, you refer to the first Lemma of the first Section of the first Book of Sir *Isaac*'s Principles. I answer, that if $a$ and $b$ are real quantities, then $ab$ is something, and consequently makes a real difference: but if they are nothing, then the Rectangles whereof they are coefficients become nothing likewise: and consequently the *momentum* or *incrementum*, whether Sir *Isaac*'s or mine, are in that Case nothing at all. As for the abovementioned Lemma, which you refer to, and which you wish I had consulted sooner, both for my own sake and for yours; I tell you I had long since consulted and considered it. But I very much doubt whether you have sufficiently considered that Lemma, it's Demonstration and it's Consequences. For, however that way of reasoning may do in the Method of *exhaustions*, where quantities less than assignable are regarded as nothing; yet for a Fluxionist writing about momentums, to argue that quantities must be equal because they have no assignable difference, seems the most injudicious Step that could be taken: it is directly demolishing the very Doctrine you would defend. For it will thence follow, that all homogeneous momentums are equal, and consequently the velocities, mutations, or fluxions proportional thereto, are all likewise equal. There is, therefore, only one proportion of equality throughout, which at once overthrows the whole System you undertake to defend. Your moments (I say) not being themselves assignable quantities, their differences cannot be assignable: and if this be true, by that way of reasoning it will follow, they are all equal, upon which Supposition you cannot make one Step in the Method of Fluxions. It appears from hence, how unjustly you blame me (*P.* 32) for omitting to give any Account of that first Section of the first Book of the *Principia*, wherein (you say) the Foundation of the Method of Fluxions is geometrically demonstrated and largely explained, and difficulties and objections against it are clearly solved. All which is so far from being true, that the very first and fundamental Lemma of that Section is incompatible with, and subversive of the doctrine of Fluxions. And, indeed, who sees not that a Demonstration *ad absurdum more veterum* proceeding on a Supposition, that every difference must be some given quantity, cannot be admitted in, or consist with, a method, wherein Quantities, less than any given, are supposed really to exist, and be capable of division?

XXXIII. The next point you undertake to defend is that method for obtaining a rule to find the Fluxion of any Power of a flowing Quantity, which is delivered in the introduction to the Quadratures, and considered in the Analyst.[5] And here the question between us is, whether I have rightly represented the sense of those words, *evanescant jam augmenta illa*, in rendering them, let the increments vanish *i.e.* let the increments be nothing, or let there be no increments? This you deny, but, as your manner is, instead of giving a reason you declaim. I, on the contrary affirm, the increments must be understood to be quite gone and absolutely nothing at all. My reason is, because without that supposition you can never bring the quantity or expression

$$x^n + nox^{n-1} + \frac{nn-n}{2}oox^{n-2} + \&c.$$

down to $nx^{n-1}$, the very thing aimed at by supposing the evanescence. Say whether this be not the truth of the case? Whether the former expression is not to be reduced to the latter? And whether this can possibly be done so long as *o* is supposed a real Quantity? I cannot indeed say you are scrupulous about your affirmations, and yet I believe that even you will not affirm this; it being most evident, that the product of two real quantities is something real; and that nothing real can be rejected either according to the ἀκρίβεια of Geometry, or according to Sir *Isaac*'s own Principles; for the truth of which I appeal to all who know any thing of these matters. Further by *evanescant* must either be meant let them (the increments) vanish and become nothing, in the obvious sense, or let them become infinitely small. But that this latter is not Sir *Isaac*'s sense is evident from his own words in the very same page, that is, in the last of the Introduction to the Quadratures, where he expressly saith *volui ostendere quod in methodo fluxionum non opus sit figuras infinite parvas in geometriam introducere*. Upon the whole, you

---

[5] Sect. 13, 14, &c.

seem to have considered this affair so very superficially, as greatly to confirm me in the opinion, you are so angry with, to wit, that Sir *Isaac*'s followers are much more eager in applying his method, than accurate in examining his principles. You raise a dust about evanescent augments which may perhaps amuse and amaze your Reader, but I am much mistaken if it ever instructs or enlightens him. For, to come to the point, those evanescent augments either are real quantities, or they are not. If you say they are; I desire to know, how you get rid of the rejectaneous quantity? If you say they are not; you indeed get rid of those quantities in the composition whereof they are coefficients; but then you are of the same opinion with me, which opinion you are pleased to call (*P.* 58) "a most palpable, inexcusable, and unpardonable blunder," although it be a Truth most palpably evident.

XXXIV. Nothing I say can be plainer to any impartial Reader, than that by the Evanescence of augments, in the above-cited passage, Sir *Isaac* means their being actually reduced to nothing. But to put it out of all doubt, that this is the truth, and to convince even you, who shew so little disposition to be convinced, I desire you to look into his *Analysis per æquationes infinitas* (*P.* 20) where, in his preparation for demonstrating the first rule for the squaring of simple Curves, you will find that on a parallel occasion, speaking of an augment which is supposed to vanish, he interprets the word *evanescere* by *esse nihil*. Nothing can be plainer than this, which at once destroys your defence. And yet, plain as it is, I despair of making you acknowledge it; though I am sure you feel it, and the Reader if he useth his eyes must see it. The words *Evanescere sive esse nihil* do (to use your own expression) stare us in the face. Lo! This is what you call (*P.* 56) "so great, so unaccountable, so horrid, so truly *Boeotian* a blunder" that, according to you, it was not possible Sir Isaac Newton could be guilty of it. For the future, I advise you to be more sparing of hard words: Since, as you incautiously deal them about, they may chance to light on your friends as well as your adversaries. As for my part, I shall not retaliate. It is sufficient to say you are mistaken. But I can easily pardon your mistakes. Though, indeed, you tell me on this very occasion, that I must expect no quarter from Sir *Isaac*'s followers. And I tell you that I neither expect nor desire any. My aim is truth. My reasons I have given. Confute them, if you can. But think not to overbear me either with authorities or harsh words. The latter will recoil upon your selves: The former in a matter of science are of no weight with indifferent Readers; and as for Bigots, I am not concerned about what they say or think.

XXXV. In the next place you proceed to declaim upon the following passage taken from the seventeenth section of the Analyst. "Considering the various arts and devices used by the great author of the fluxionary method: in how many lights he placeth his Fluxions: and in what different ways he attempts to demonstrate the same point: One would be inclined to think, he was himself suspicious of the justness of his own demonstrations." This passage you complain of as very hard usage of Sir *Isaac Newton*. You declaim copiously, and endeavour to show that placing the same point in various lights is of great use to explain it; which you illustrate with much Rhetoric. But the fault of that passage is not the hard usage it contains: But on the contrary, that it is too modest, and not so full and expressive of my sense, as perhaps it should have been. Would you like it better if I should say, the various *inconsistent* accounts, which this great author gives of his momentums and his fluxions, may convince every intelligent Reader that he had no clear and steady notions of them, without which there can be no demonstration? I own frankly that I see no clearness or consistence in them. You tell me indeed, in *Miltonic* verse that the fault is in my own eyes,

*So thick a drop serene has quench'd their orbs Or dim suffusion veil'd.*

at the same time you acknowledge your self obliged for those various lights, which have enabled you to understand his

Doctrine. But as for me who do not understand it, you insult me saying: "For God's sake what is it you are offended at, who do not still understand him?" May not I answer, that I am offended for this very reason; because I cannot understand him or make sense of what he says? You say to me, that I am all in the dark. I acknowledge it, and intreat you who see so clearly to help me out.

XXXVI. You Sir with the bright eyes, be pleased to tell me, whether Sir *Isaac's* momentum be a finite quantity, or an infinitesimal, or a mere limit? If you say a finite quantity: Be pleased to reconcile this with what he saith in the Scholium of the second Lemma of the first Section of the first book of his Principles: *Cave intelligas quantitates magnitudine determinatas, sed cogita semper diminuendas sine limite.* If you say, an infinitesimal: reconcile this with what is said in the Introduction to the Quadratures: *Volui ostendere quod in methodo Fluxionum non opus sit figuras infinite parvas in Geometriam introducere.* If you should say, it is a mere limit, be pleased to reconcile this with what we find in the first case of the second Lemma in the second book of his Principles: *Ubi de lateribus* A *et* B *deerant momentorum dimidia,* &c. where the moments are supposed to be divided. I should be very glad, a person of such a luminous intellect would be so good as to explain, whether by Fluxions we are to understand the nascent or evanescent quantities themselves, or their motions, or their Velocities, or simply their proportions: and having interpreted them in what sense you will, that you would then condescend to explain the Doctrine of second, third, and fourth Fluxions, and shew it to be consistent with common sense if you can. You seem to be very sanguine when you express your self in the following terms: "I do assure you, Sir, from my own Experience, and that of many others whom I could name that the Doctrine may be clearly conceived and distinctly comprehended" (*P.* 31). And it may be uncivil not to believe what you so solemnly affirm, from your own experience. But I must needs own, I should be better satisfied of this, if, instead of entertaining us with your Rhetoric, you would vouchsafe to reconcile those difficulties, and explain those obscure points abovementioned. If either you, or any one of those many whom you could name, will but explain to others what you so clearly conceive your selves, I give you my word that several will be obliged to you who, I may venture to say, understand those matters no more than my self. But, if I am not mistaken, you and your friends will modestly decline this task.

XXXVII. I have long ago done what you so often exhort me to do, diligently read and considered the several accounts of this Doctrine given by the great Author in different parts of his writings: any upon the whole I could never make it out to be consistent and intelligible. I was even led to say, that "one would be inclined to think, He was himself suspicious of the justness of his own demonstrations: and that he was not enough pleased with any one notion steadily to adhere to it." After which I added, "Thus much is plain that he owned himself satisfied concerning certain points, which nevertheless he could not undertake to demonstrate to others." See the seventeenth section of the Analyst. It is one thing when a Doctrine is placed in various lights: and another, when the principles and notions are shifted. When new devices are introduced and substituted for others, a Doctrine instead of being illustrated may be explained away. Whether there be not something of this in the present case I appeal to the writings of the Great Author. His *methodus rationum primarum et ultimarum*, His second Lemma in the second book of his Principles, his Introduction and Treatise of the Quadrature of Curves. In all which it appears to me, there is not one uniform doctrine explained and carried throughout the whole, but rather sundry inconsistent accounts of this new method, which still grows more dark and confused the more it is handled: I could not help thinking, the greatest genius might lye under the influence of false principles; and where the object and notions were exceeding obscure, he might possibly distrust even his own demonstrations. "At least thus much seemed plain, that Sir *Isaac* had sometime owned himself satisfied, where he could not demonstrate to others." In proof whereof I mentioned his letter to Mr. *Collins*; Hereupon you tell me: "there is a great deal of difference between saying, I cannot undertake to prove a thing, and I will not undertake it." But in answer to this, I desire you will be pleased to consider, that I was not making a precise extract out of that letter, in which the very words of Sir *Isaac* should alone be inserted. But I made my own remark and inference, from what I remembered to have read in that letter; where, speaking of a certain mathematical matter, Sir *Isaac* expresseth himself, in the following terms: "It is plain to me by the fountain I draw it from; though I will not undertake to prove it to others." Now whether my inference may not be fairly drawn from those words of Sir *Isaac Newton*; and whether the difference as to the sense be so great between *will* and *can* in that particular case, I leave to be determined by the Reader.

XXXVIII. In the next paragraph you talk big but prove nothing. You speak of driving out of intrenchments, of sallying and attacking and carrying by assault; of slight and untenable works, of a new-raised and undisciplined militia, and of veteran regular troops. Need the Reader be a Mathematician to see the vanity of this paragraph? After this you employ (*P.* 65) your usual colouring, and represent the great Author of the Method of Fluxions "as a Good old Gentleman fast asleep, and snoring in his easy chair; while dame Fortune is bringing him her apron full of beautiful theorems and problems, which he never knows or thinks of." This you would have pass for a consequence of my notions. But I appeal to all those who are ever so little knowing in such matters, whether there are not divers fountains of Experiment, Induction, and Analogy, whence a man may derive and satisfy himself concerning the truth of many points in Mathematics and Mechanical Philosophy, although the proofs thereof afforded by the modern Analysis should not amount to demonstration? I further appeal to the conscience of all the most profound Mathematicians, whether they can, with perfect acquiescence of mind free from all scruple, apply any proposition merely upon the strength of a Demonstration involving second or third Fluxions, without the aid of any such experiment or analogy or collateral proof whatsoever? Lastly, I appeal to the Reader's own heart, whether he cannot clearly conceive a medium between being fast asleep and demonstrating? But you will have it, that I represent Sir *Isaac*'s Conclusions as coming out right, because one errour is compensated by another contrary and equal errour, which perhaps he never knew himself nor thought of: that by a twofold mistake he arrives though not at science yet at Truth: that he proceeds blindfold, &c. All which is untruly said by you, who have misapplied to Sir *Isaac* what was intended for the Marquis de l'*Hospital* and his followers, for no other end (as I can see) but that you may have an opportunity, to draw that ingenious portraiture of Sir *Isaac Newton* and Dame Fortune, as will be manifest to whoever reads the Analyst.

XXXIX. You tell me (*P.* 70), if I think fit to persist in asserting, "that this affair of a double errour is entirely a new discovery of my own, which Sir *Isaac* and his followers never knew or thought of, that you have unquestionable evidence to convince me to the contrary, and that all his followers are already apprised, that this very objection of mine was long since foreseen, and clearly and fully removed by Sir *Isaac Newton* in the first section of the first book of his *Principia*." All which I do as strongly deny as you affirm. And I do aver, that this is an unquestionable proof of the matchless contempt which you, *Philalethes*, have for Truth. And I do here publickly call upon you, to produce that evidence which you pretend to have, and to make good that fact which you so confidently affirm. And, at the same time, I do assure the Reader that you never will, nor can.

XL. If you defend Sir *Isaac*'s notions as delivered in his *Principia*, it must be on the rigorous foot of rejecting nothing, neither admitting nor casting away infinitely small quantities. If you defend the Marquis, whom you also style your Master, it must be on the foot of admitting that there are infinitesimals, that they may be rejected, that they are nevertheless real quantities, and themselves infinitely subdivisible. But you seem to have grown giddy with passion, and in the heat of controversy to have mistaken and forgot your part. I beseech you, Sir, to consider, that the Marquis (whom alone, and not Sir *Isaac* this double errour in finding the subtangent doth concern) rejects indeed infinitesimals, but not on the foot that you do, to wit, their being inconsiderable in practical Geometry or mixed Mathematics. But he rejects them in the accuracy of Speculative Knowledge: in which respect there may be great Logical errours, although there should be no sensible mistake in practice: which, it seems, is what you cannot comprehend. He rejects them likewise in vertue of a Postulatum, which I venture to call rejecting them without ceremony. And though he inferreth a conclusion accurately true, yet he doth it, contrary to the rules of Logic, from inaccurate and false premises. And how this comes about, I have at large explained in the Analyst, and shewed in that particular case of Tangents, that the Rejectaneous Quantity might have been a finite quantity of any given magnitude, and yet the conclusion have come out exactly the same way; and consequently, that the truth of this method doth not depend on the reason assigned by the Marquis, to wit, the *postulatum* for throwing away Infinitesimals, and therefore that he and his follows acted blindfold, as not knowing the true reason for the conclusions coming out accurately right, which I shew to have been the effect of a double errour.

XLI. This is the truth of the matter, which you shamefully misrepresent and declaim upon, to no sort of purpose but to amuse and mislead your Reader. For which conduct of yours throughout your remarks, you will pardon me if I cannot otherwise account, than from a secret hope that the Reader of your defence would never read the Analyst. If he doth, He cannot but see what an admirable Method you take to defend your cause: How instead of justifying the Reasoning, the Logic or the Theory of the case specified, which is the real point, you discourse of sensible and practical errours: And how all this is a manifest imposition upon the Reader. He must needs see that I have expressly said, "I have no controversy except only about your Logic and method: that I consider how you demonstrate; what objects you are conversant about; and whether you conceive them clearly?" That I have often expressed my self to the same effect desiring the Reader to remember, "that I am only concerned about the way of coming at your theorems, whether it be legitimate or illegitimate, clear or obscure, scientific or tentative: That I have on this very occasion, to prevent all possibility of mistake, repeated and insisted that I consider the Geometrical Analyst as a Logician *i.e.* so far forth as he reasons and argues; and his mathematical conclusions not in themselves but in their premises; not as true or false, useful or insignificant, but as derived from such principles, and by such inferences."[6] You affirm (and indeed what can you not affirm?) that the difference between the true subtangent and that found without any compensation is absolutely nothing at all. I profess my self of a contrary opinion. My reason is because nothing cannot be divided into parts. But this difference is capable of being divided into any, or into more than any given number of parts; For the truth of which consult the Marquis de l'*Hospital*. And, be the errour in fact or in practice ever so small, it will not thence follow that the errour in Reasoning, which is what I am alone concerned about, is one whit the less, it being evident that a man may reason most absurdly about the minutest things.

XLII. Pray answer me fairly, once for all, whether it be your opinion that whatsoever is little and inconsiderable enough to be rejected without inconvenience in practice, the same may in like manner be safely rejected and overlooked in Theory and Demonstration. if you say *no*, it will then follow, that all you have been saying here and elsewhere, about yards and inches and decimal fractions, setting forth and insisting on the extreme

---

[6] 'Analyst,' Sect. 20.

smallness of the rejectaneous quantity, is quite foreign to the argument, and only a piece of skill to impose upon your Reader. If you say *yes*, it follows that you then give up at once all the orders of Fluxions and Infinitesimal Differences; and so most imprudently turn all your sallies and attacks and Veterans to your own overthrow. If the Reader is of my mind, he will despair of ever seeing you get clear of this dilemma. The points in controversy have been so often and so distinctly noted in the Analyst, that I very much wonder how you could mistake if you had no mind to mistake. It is very plain, if you are in earnest, that you neither understand me nor your Masters. And what shall we think of other ordinary Analysts, when it shall be found that even you, who, like a Champion step forth to defend their principles, have not considered them?

XLIII. The impartial reader is entreated to remark throughout your whole performance how confident you are in asserting and withall how modest in proving or explaining: How frequent it is with you to employ Figures and Tropes instead of Reasons: How many difficulties proposed in the Analyst are discreetly overlooked by you, and what strange work you make with the rest: How grossly you mistake and misrepresent, and how little you practise the advice which you so liberally bestow. Believe me Sir, I had long and maturely considered the principles of the modern Analysis, before I ventured to publish my thoughts thereupon in the Analyst. And since the publication thereof, I have my self freely conversed with Mathematicians of all ranks, and some of the ablest Professors, as well as made it my business to be informed of the Opinions of others, being very desirous to hear what could be said towards clearing my difficulties or answering my objections. But though you are not afraid or ashamed, to represent the Analysts as very clear and uniform in their Conception of these matters, yet I do solemnly affirm (and several of themselves know it to be true) that I found no harmony or agreement among them, but the reverse thereof, the greatest dissonance and even contrariety of Opinions, employed to explain what after all seemed inexplicable.

XLIV. Some fly to proportions between nothings. Some reject quantities because infinitesimal. Others allow only finite quantities, and reject them because inconsiderable. Others place the method of Fluxions on a foot with that of *exhaustions*, and admit nothing new therein. Some maintain the clear conception of Fluxions. Others hold they can demonstrate about things incomprehensible. Some would prove the Algorism of Fluxions by *reductio ad absurdum*; others *a priori*. Some hold the evanescent increments to be real quantities, some to be nothings, some to be limits. As many Men, so many minds: each differing one from another, and all from Sir *Isaac Newton*. Some plead inaccurate expressions in the great Author, whereby they would draw him to speak their sense, not considering that if he meant as they do, he could not want words to express his meaning. Others are magisterial and positive, say they are satisfied, and that is all, not considering that we, who deny Sir *Isaac Newton*'s Authority, shall not submit to that of his Disciples. Some insist, that the Conclusions are true, and therefore the principles, not considering what hath been largely said in the Analyst[7] on that head. Lastly several (and those none of the meanest) frankly owned the objections to be unanswerable. All which I mention by way of Antidote to your false Colours: and that the unprejudiced Inquirer after Truth may see, it is not without foundation, that I call on the celebrated Mathematicians of the present Age to clear up these obscure Analytics, and concur in giving to the publick some consistent and intelligible account of the principles of their great Master: for if they do not, I believe the World will take it for granted that they cannot.

XLV. Having gone through your defence of the British Mathematicians, I find in the next place, that you attack me on a

---

[7] *Sect.* 19, 20. &c.

point of Metaphysics, with what success the Reader will determine. I had upon another occasion many years ago wrote against Abstract general Ideas.[8] In opposition to which, you declare your self to adhere to the vulgar opinion, that neither Geometry nor any other general Science can subsist without general Ideas (*P. 74*). This implies that I hold there are no general Ideas. But I hold the direct contrary, that there are indeed general Ideas, but not formed by abstraction in the manner set forth by Mr. *Locke*. To me it is plain, there is no consistent Idea, the likeness whereof may not really exist. Whatsoever therefore is said to be somewhat which cannot exist, the Idea thereof must be inconsistent. Mr *Locke* acknowledgeth it doth require Pains and Skill to form his general Idea of a triangle. He farther expressly saith, it must be neither oblique nor rectangular, neither equilateral, equicrural, nor scalenum; but all and none of these of these at once. He also saith, it is an idea wherein some parts of several different and inconsistent Ideas are put together.[9] All this looks very like a Contradiction. But to put the matter past dispute, it must be noted, that he affirms it to be somewhat imperfect that cannot exist; consequently the Idea thereof is impossible or inconsistent.

XLVI. I desire to know, whether it is not possible for any thing to exist, which doth not include a contradiction: And if it is, whether we may not infer, that what may not possibly exist, the same doth include a contradiction: I further desire to know, whether the reader can frame a distinct idea of anything that includes a contradiction? For my part, I cannot, nor consequently of the abovementioned triangle; Though you (you it seems know better than my self what I can do) are pleased to assure me of the contrary. Again, I ask whether that, which it is above the power of man to form a compleat idea of, may not be called incomprehensible? And whether the Reader can frame a compleat

---

[8] *Introduction to a Treatise concerning the Principles of Human Knowledge printed in the Year MDCCX.*
[9] *Essay on Humane Understanding*, b. iv, c. vii, § ix.

idea of this imperfect impossible triangle? And if not, whether it doth not follow that it is incomprehensible? It should seem, that a distinct aggregate of a few consistent parts was nothing so difficult to conceive or impossible to exist; and that, therefore, your Comment must be wide of the Author's meaning. You give me to understand (*P.* 82) that this account of a general triangle was a trap which Mr. *Locke* set to catch fools. Who is caught therein let the Reader judge.

XLVII. It is Mr. *Locke*'s opinion, that every general name stands for a general abstract idea, which prescinds from the species or individuals comprehended under it. Thus, for example, according to him, the general name *Colour* stands for an idea, which is neither Blue, Red, Green, nor any particular colour, but somewhat distinct and abstracted from them all. To me it seems the word *Colour* is only a more general name applicable to all and each of the particular colours; while the other specific names, as Blue, Red, Green, and the like are each restrained to a more limited signification. The same can be said of the word *Triangle.* Let the Reader judge whether this be not the case; and whether he can distinctly frame such an idea of colour as shall prescind from all the species thereof, or of a triangle which shall answer Mr. *Locke*'s account, prescinding and abstracting from all the particular sorts of triangles, in the manner aforesaid.

XLVIII. I entreat my Reader to think. For if he doth not, he may be under some influence from your confident and positive way of talking. But any one who thinks may, if I mistake not, plainly perceive that you are deluded, as it often happens, by mistaking the terms for ideas. Nothing is easier, than to define in terms or words that which is incomprehensible in idea, forasmuch as any words can be either separated or joined as you please, but ideas always cannot. It is as easy to say a round square as an oblong square, though the former be inconceivable. If the Reader will but take a little care to distinguish between the Definition and the Idea, between words or expressions and the conceptions of the mind, he will judge of the truth of what I now advance, and clearly perceive how far you are mistaken, in attempting to illustrate Mr. *Locke*'s Doctrine, and where your mistake lies. Or, if the Reader is minded to make short work, he needs only at once to try, whether laying aside the words he can frame in his mind the idea of an impossible triangle; upon which trial the issue of this dispute may be fairly put. This doctrine of abstract general ideas seemed to me a capital errour, productive of numberless difficulties and disputes, that runs not only throughout Mr. *Locke*'s book but through most parts of Learning. Consequently, my animadversions thereupon were not an effect of being inclined to carp or cavil at a single passage, as you would wrongfully insinuate, but proceeded from a love of Truth, and a desire to banish, so far as in me lay, false principles and wrong ways of thinking, without respect of persons. And indeed, though you and other Party-men are violently attached to your respective Masters, yet I, who profess my self only attached to Truth, see no reason why I may not as freely animadvert on Mr. *Locke* or Sir *Isaac Newton*, as they would on *Aristotle* or *Descartes*. Certainly the more extensive the influence of any Errour, and the greater the authority which supports it, the more it deserves to be considered and detected by sincere Inquirers after Knowledge.

XLIX. In the close of your performance, you let me understand, that your Zeal for Truth and the reputation of your Masters have occasioned your reprehending me with the utmost freedom. And it must be owned you have shewn a singular talent therein. But I am comforted under the severity of your reprehensions, when I consider the weakness of your arguments, which, were they as strong as your reproofs, could leave no doubt in the mind of the Reader concerning the matters in dispute between us. As it is, I leave him to reflect and examine by your light, how clearly he is enabled to conceive a fluxion, or a fluxion of a fluxion, a part infinitely small subdivided into an infinity of parts, a nascent or evanescent increment, that which is neither something nor nothing, a triangle formed in a point, velocity without motion, and the rest of those *arcana* of the modern Analysis. To conclude, I had some thoughts of advising you how to conduct your self for the future, in return for the advice you have so freely imparted to me: but, as you think it becomes me rather to inform my self than instruct others, I shall, for my farther information, take leave to propose a few Queries to those learned Gentlemen of *Cambridge*, whom you associate with your self, and represent as being equally surprised at the tendency of my Analyst.

L. I desire to know, whether those who can neither demonstrate nor conceive the principles of the modern Analysis, and yet give in to it, may not be justly said to have Faith, and be styled believers of mysteries? Whether it is impossible to find among the Physicians, mechanical Philosophers, Mathematicians, and Philomathematicians of the present age, some such Believers, who yet deride Christians for their belief of Mysteries? Whether with such men it is not a fair, reasonable, and legitimate method to use the *Argumentum ad Hominem*? And being so, whether it ought to surprise either Christians or Scholars? Whether in an age wherein so many pretenders to science attack the Christian Religion, we may not be allowed to make reprisals, in order to shew that the Irreligion of those men is not to be presumed an effect of deep and just thinking? Whether an attempt to detect false reasonings, and remedy defects in Mathematics, ought to be ill received by Mathematicians? Whether the introducing more easy methods and more intelligible principles in any science should be discountenanced? Whether there may not be fair objections as well as cavils? And whether to inquire diligently into the meaning of terms and the proof of propositions, not excepting against anything without assigning a reason, nor affecting to mistake the signification of words, or stick at an expression where the sense was clear, but considering the subject in all lights, sincerely endeavouring to find out any sense or meaning whatsoever, candidly setting forth what seems obscure and what fallacious, and calling upon those, who profess the knowledge of such matters, to explain them, whether I say such a proceeding can be justly called cavilling? Whether there be an *ipse dixit* erected? And if so, when, where, by whom, and upon what Authority? Whether even where Authority was to take place, one might not hope the Mathematics, at least, would be excepted? Whether the chief end, in making Mathematics so considerable a part of Academical Education, be not to form in the minds of young Students habits of just and exact Reasoning? And whether the study of abstruse and subtile matters can conduce to this end, unless they are well understood, examined, and sifted to the bottom? Whether, therefore, the bringing Geometrical demonstrations to the severest test of Reason should be reckoned a discouragement to the studies of any learned Society? Whether to separate the clear parts of things from the obscure, to distinguish the real Principles whereon Truths rest, and whence they are derived, and to proportion the just measures of assent according to the various degrees of evidence, be a useless or unworthy undertaking? Whether the making more of an argument than it will bear, and placing it in an undue rank of evidence, be not the likely way to disparage it? Whether it may not be of some use, to provoke and stir up the learned professors to explain a part of Mathematical Learning, which is acknowledged to be most profound, difficult, and obscure, and at the same time set forth by *Philalethes* and many others, as the greatest instance that has ever been given of the extent of humane abilities? Whether for the sake of a Great man's discoveries, we must adopt his errours? Lastly, whether in an age wherein all other principles are canvassed with the utmost freedom, the principles of Fluxions are to be alone excepted?

# An Appendix Concerning Mr. *Walton*'s Vindication Of Sir Isaac Newton's Principles of Fluxions

I. I had no sooner considered the performance of *Philalethes*, but Mr. *Walton*'s Vindication of Fluxions was put into my hands. As this *Dublin* professor gleans after the *Cantabrigian*, only endeavouring to translate a few passages from Sir *Isaac Newton*'s *Principia*, and enlarge on a hint or two of *Philalethes*, he deserves no particular notice. It may suffice to advertise the Reader, that the foregoing defence, contains a full and explicit answer to Mr. *Walton*, as he will find, if he thinks it worth his pains to read what this Gentleman hath written, and compare it therewith: Particularly with Sect. 18, 20, 30, 32, 33, 34, 35, 36, 43. It is not, I am sure, worth mine to repeat the same things, or confute the same notions twice over, in mere regard to a writer who hath copied even the manners of *Philalethes*, and whom in answering the other I have, if I am not much mistaken, sufficiently answered.

II. Mr. *Walton* touches on the same points that the other had touched upon before him. He pursues a hint which the other had given[10], about Sir *Isaac*'s first Section concerning the *Rationes primae et ultimae*. He discreetly avoids, like the other, to say one syllable of second, third, or fourth Fluxions, and of divers other points mentioned in the Analyst, about all which I observe in him a most prudent and profound silence. And yet he very modestly gives his Reader to understand, that he is able to clear up all difficulties and objections, that have ever been made (*P.* 5). Mr. *Walton* in the beginning, like *Philalethes*, from a particular case makes a general inference, supposing that Infidelity to be imputed to Mathematicians in general, which I suppose only in the person to whom the Analyst was addressed, and certain other persons of the same mind with him. Whether this extraordinary way of reasoning be the cause or effect of his passion, I know not: But before I had got to the end of his Vindication, I ceased to be

---

[10] *Philalethes*, p. 32.

surprized at his Logic and his temper in the beginning. The double errour, which in the Analyst was plainly meant to belong to others, he with *Philalethes* (whose very oversight he adopts) supposeth to have been ascribed to Sir *Isaac Newton* (P. 36). And this writer also, as well as the *Cantabrigian*, must needs take upon him to explain the motive of my writing against Fluxions: which he gives out, with great assurance, to have been, because Sir *Isaac Newton* had presumed to interpose in Prophecies and Revelations, and to decide in religious affairs (P. 4) which is so far from being true, that, on the contrary, I have a high value for those learned remains of that Great Man, whose original and free Genius is an eternal reproach to that tribe of followers, who are always imitating, but never resemble him. This specimen of Mr. *Walton*'s truth will be a warning to the Reader to use his own eyes, and in obscure points never to trust the Gentleman's Candour, who dares to misrepresent the plainest.

III. I was thinking to have said no more concerning this Author's performance, but lest he should imagine himself too much neglected, I entreat the Reader to have the patience to peruse it; and if he finds any one point of the doctrine of Fluxions cleared up, or any one objection in the Analyst answered, or so much as fairly stated, let him then make his compliments to the Author. But, if he can no more make sense of what this Gentleman has written than I can, he will need no answer to it. Nothing is easier, than for a man to translate or copy, or compose a plausible discourse of some pages in technical terms, whereby he shall make a shew of saying somewhat, although neither the Reader nor himself understand one Tittle of it. Whether this be the case of Mr. *Walton*, and whether he understands either Sir *Isaac Newton*, or me, or himself, (whatever I may think) I shall not take it upon me to say. But one thing I know, that many an unmeaning Speech passeth for significant by the mere assurance of the Speaker, till he cometh to be catechised upon it; and then the truth sheweth it self. This Vindicator, indeed, by his dissembling nine parts in ten of the difficulties proposed in the

Analyst, sheweth no inclination to be catechised by me. But his Scholars have a right to be informed. I therefore, recommend it to them, not to be imposed on by hard words and magisterial assertions, but carefully to pry into his sense, and sift his meaning, and particularly to insist on a distinct answer to the following Questions.

IV. Let them ask him, whether he can conceive velocity without motion, or motion without extension, or extension without magnitude? If he answers that he can, let him teach them to do the same. If he cannot, let him be asked, how he reconciles the idea of a Fluxion which he gives (*P.* 13,) with common sense? Again, let him be asked, whether nothing be not the product of nothing multiplied by something? And if so, when the difference between the Gnomon and the sum of the rectangles[11] vanisheth, whether the rectangles themselves do not also vanish? *i.e.* when $ab$ is nothing, whether $Ab + Ba$ be not also nothing? *i.e.* whether the momentum of $AB$ be not nothing? Let him then be asked, what his momentums are good for, when they are thus brought to nothing? Again, I wish he were asked to explain the difference, between a magnitude infinitely small and a magnitude infinitely diminished. If he saith there is no difference: Then let him be farther asked, how he dares to explain the method of Fluxions, by the *Ratio* of magnitudes infinitely diminished (*P.* 9), when Sir *Isaac Newton* hath expressly excluded all consideration of quantities infinitely small?[12] If this able vindicator should say that quantities infinitely diminished are nothing at all, and consequently that, according to him, the first and last *Ratio*'s are proportions between nothings, let him be desired to make sense of this, or explain what he means by *proportion between nothings*. If he should say the ultimate proportions are the *Ratio*'s of mere limits, then let him be asked how the limits of lines can be proportioned or divided? After all, who knows but this Gentleman, who hath already complained of me for an

---

[11] See *Vindication*, p. 17.
[12] See his *Introduction to the Quadratures*.

uncommon way of treating Mathematics and Mathematicians (*P.* 5), may (as well as the *Cantabrigian*) cry out *Spain* and the *Inquisition*, when he finds himself thus closely pursued and beset with Interrogatories? That we may not, therefore seem too hard on an innocent man, who probably meant nothing, but was betray'd by following another into difficulties and straits that he was not aware of, I shall propose one single expedient, by which his Disciples (whom it most concerns) may soon satisfy themselves, whether this Vindicator really understands what he takes upon him to vindicate. It is in short, that they would ask him to explain the second, third or fourth Fluxions upon his Principles. Be this the Touchstone of his vindication. If he can do it, I shall own my self much mistaken: If he cannot, it will be evident that he was much mistaken in himself, when he presumed to defend Fluxions without so much as knowing what they are. So having put the merits of the cause on this issue, I leave him to be tried by his Scholars.

www.ingramcontent.com/pod-product-compliance
Lightning Source LLC
Chambersburg PA
CBHW071752090426
42738CB00011B/2658